Sirtfood Diet mastery

Mouthwatering Recipes for a Rapid Weight Loss, A Meal Plan to Turn On your Skinny Gene, Burn Fat, Boost Energy, and Reset Metabolism in 7 days

Lisa T. Oliver

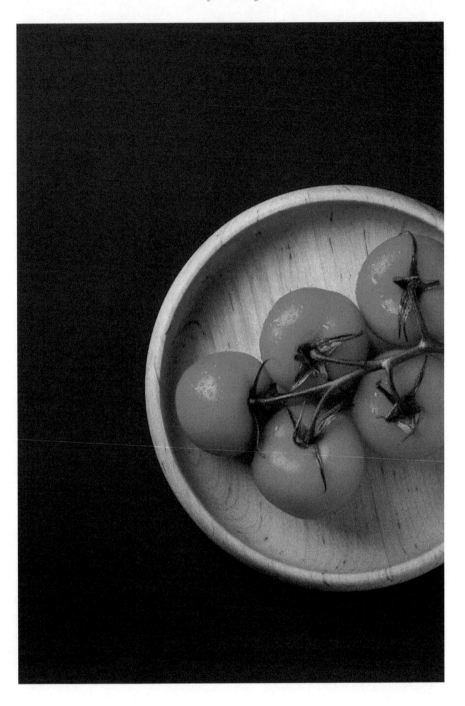

Table Of Contents

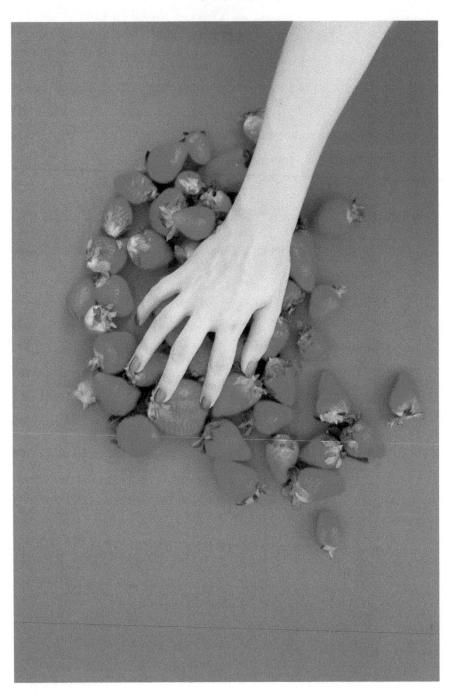

Introduction

The Sirtfood Diet, launched in 2016, has been a trending topic for a while now, with people following the diet very strictly. The creators of the diet suggest that these foods function by activating proteins in the body, referred to as sirtuins. The idea is that sirtuins protect body cells from dying when subjected to stress and regulate metabolism, inflammation, and aging. Sirtuins also boost the body's metabolism and affect its ability to burn fat, providing a weight loss of about seven pounds in a week while retaining muscle.

What Are Sirtfoods?

Sirtuins refer to a protein class that has been proven to regulate the metabolism of fat and glucose. According to research, sirtuins also have a significant impact on aging, inflammation, and cell death.

By consuming foods rich in sirtuins like cocoa, kale, and parsley, you stimulate your skinny gene pathway and lose fat faster.

About the Sirtfood Diet

The Sirtfood Diet plan considers that some foods activate your "skinny gene" and can make you lose about seven pounds in about a week.Certain foods, such as dark chocolate, kale, and wine, contain polyphenols, a natural chemical that imitates exercise and fasting and affects the body. Other sirtfoods include cinnamon, red onions, and turmeric. These trigger the sirtuins' pathway and start weight loss. There is scientific evidence to support this too. The impact of weight loss is higher in the first week. The Sirtfood Diet mainly consists of plant-based foods that are rich in sirtuins to trigger fat loss. The diet is divided into two phases, which can be repeated continuously.The first phase is three days of living on 1000 calories and four days of 1500 calories with lots of green juices.

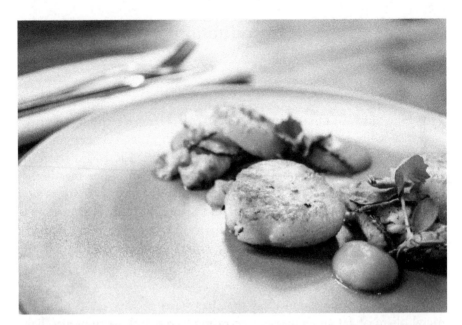

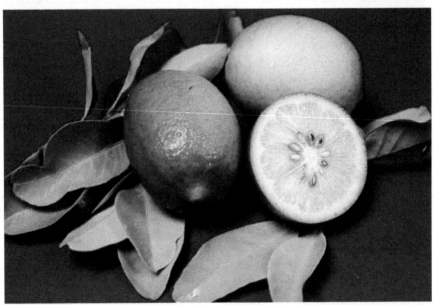

CHAPTER 1

Breakfast

1. Buckwheat Superfood Muesli

Preparation Time: 10 minutes

Cooking Time: 0 minutes

Servings: 4

Ingredients:

- 20g buckwheat pieces

- 10g buckwheat puffs

- 15g coconut pieces or parched coconut

- 40g Medjool dates, hollowed and cleaved

- 15g walnuts, cleaved

- 10g cocoa nibs

- 100g strawberries, hulled and cleaved

- 100g plain Greek yogurt (or veggie lover elective, for example, soy or coconut yogurt)

Directions:

Blend the entirety of the above Ingredients: together (forget about the strawberries and yogurt if not serving straight away).

Notes

If you need to make this in mass or set it up the previous night, just join the dry Ingredients: and store it in an impenetrable holder. All you have to do the following day is include the strawberries and yogurt, and it is all set.

2.   Buckwheat Pancakes With Strawberries, Dark Chocolate Sauce, And Crushed Walnuts

Preparation Time: 10 minutes

Cooking Time: 40 minutes

Servings: 4

Ingredients:

For the flapjacks, you will require:

•   350ml milk

•   150g buckwheat flour

•   1 huge egg

•   1 tbsp. additional virgin olive oil, for cooking

For the chocolate sauce

•   100g dull chocolate (85 percent cocoa solids)

•   85ml milk

•   1 tbsp. twofold cream

•   1 tbsp. additional virgin olive oil

To serve

•   400g strawberries, hulled and cleaved

•   100g walnuts, cleaved

Directions:

To make the hotcake player, place the Ingredients' entirety: separated from the olive oil in a blender and mix until you have a smooth hitter. It ought not to be excessively thick or excessively runny. (You can store any abundance hitter in a water/air proof holder for as long as five days in your cooler. Make sure to blend a long time before utilizing once more.)

To make the chocolate sauce, soften the chocolate in a heatproof bowl over a stewing water container. When dissolved, blend in the milk, whisking thoroughly, and afterward include the twofold cream and olive oil. You can keep the sauce warm by leaving the water in the dish stewing on a shallow heat until your flapjacks are prepared.

To make the flapjacks heat a substantial bottomed griddle until it begins to smoke, including the olive oil.

Empty a portion of the player into the container's focal point. At that pointed tip, the overabundance hitter around it until you has secured the entire surface; you may need to add somewhat more player to accomplish this. You will just need to cook the hotcake for one moment, or each side of your dish is sufficiently hot.

When you can see it going dark-colored around the edges, utilize a spatula to release the flapjack around its perimeter. At that point, flip it over. Attempt to flip in one activity to abstain from breaking it.

Cook for a further moment or so on the opposite side and move to a plate.

Spot a few strawberries in the middle and move up the flapjack. Proceed until you have made the same number of pancakes as required.

Spoon over a liberal measure of sauce and sprinkle over some slashed walnuts.

You may find that your first endeavors are excessively fat or self-destruct; however, once you discover your player's consistency that works best for you and you get your method culminated, you'll be making them like an expert. Careful discipline brings about promising results right now.

3.   Blueberry Banana Pancakes With Chunky Apple Compote And Golden Turmeric Latte

Preparation Time: 10 minutes

Cooking Time: 30 minutes

Servings: 4

Ingredients:

For the Blueberry Banana Pancakes

Six bananas

Six eggs

150g moved oats

2 tsp. heating powder

¼ teaspoon salt

25g blueberries

For the Chunky Apple Compote

•   2 apples

Five dates (pitted)

1tablespoon lemon juice

1/4 teaspoon cinnamon powder

Squeeze salt

For the Golden Turmeric Latte

3 cups of coconut milk

1teaspoon turmeric powder

1teaspoon cinnamon powder

1teaspoon crude nectar

Spot of dark pepper (expands retention)

A little bit of new stripped ginger root

Place of cayenne pepper (discretionary)

Directions:

For the Blueberry Banana Pancakes

Pop the moved oats in a fast blender and heartbeat for one moment or until oat flour has its body. Tip: ensure your blender is extremely dry before doing this, or else everything will get wet!

Presently include the bananas, eggs, preparing powder, and salt to the blender and heartbeat for 2 minutes until smooth hitter structures.

Move the blend to a vast bowl and overlay in the blueberries. Leave to rest for 10 minutes while preparing powder initiates.

To make your flapjacks, include a dab of spread (this helps make them extremely tasty and fresh!) to your griddle on medium-high heat. Include a couple of spoons of the blueberry hotcake blend and fry until pleasantly brilliant on the base side. Hurl the flapjack to broil the opposite side.

For the Chunky Apple Compote

Harsh the cleave apples.

Pop everything in a nourishment processor, together with two tablespoons of water and a touch of salt—heartbeat to shape your thick apple compote. For the Golden Turmeric Latte

Mix all ingredients: in a rapid blender until smooth. Fill a little container and heat for 4 minutes over medium heat until hot, however not boiling.

Appreciate!

4.   Sirt Food Diet Green Juice Salad

Preparation Time: 10 minutes

Cooking Time: 10 minutes

Servings: 1

Ingredients

One handful rocket (arugula)

One tablespoon olive oil

Salt and pepper to taste

Two handfuls kale, sliced

One tablespoon parsley

½ green apples, sliced

Two celery sticks, sliced

1cm ginger, grated

Juice of ½ lemon

Six walnuts, halves

Directions:

Combine the lemon juice, olive oil, ginger, salt, and pepper in a jam jar and shake.

Place the kale in a large bowl and pour over the dressing. Massage the sauce into the kale for a minute. Then add all the other ingredients and mix thoroughly.

Nutrition: Calories: 290kcal| Carb: 21g| Protein: 6g| Fat: 23g|

5.　Sirt Food Diet Salmon Super Salad

Preparation Time: 10 minutes

Cooking Time: 10 minutes

Servings: 1

Ingredients

One large Medjool date, large pitted and chopped

80 g Avocado, peeled, stoned, and sliced

10g lovage or celery leaves, chopped

One tablespoon Olive oil, extra virgin

100 g Smoked salmon, slices

15g Walnuts, chopped

One tablespoon capers

1/4 juice of lemon,

50g Chicory, leaves

40g Celery, sliced

20g Red onion

10g Parsley

50g Rocket

Directions:

Place the salad leaves on a plate or in a large bowl. Mix all the ingredients and serve on top of the leaves.

Nutrition:

Energy (calories): 625 kcal

Protein: 26.76 g

Fat: 42.6 g

Carbohydrates: 40.86 g

6. Strawberry Chocolate Chip Buckwheat Pancakes

Preparation Time: 5minutes

Cooking Time: 35 minutes

Servings: 4

Ingredients

¾ cup unsweetened cashew milk (or dairy-free milk of choice)

¼ cup dark chocolate chips, dairy-free

Two tablespoons extra-virgin olive oil

One teaspoon ground cinnamon

Two tablespoons coconut sugar

One teaspoon baking powder

One tablespoon vanilla extract

½ chopped strawberries

¼ teaspoon kosher salt

1 cup buckwheat flour

One large egg

Optional Toppings:

Maple syrup

Chopped strawberries

Chocolate chips

Ground flax seeds or hemp hearts

Directions:

Heat a lightly greased skillet on medium heat.

Whisk the flour, baking powder, sugar, cinnamon, and salt together in a bowl.

Also, whisk together the milk, vanilla, oil, and eggs in another small bowl. Add the wet mixture to the dry mix and stir until combined. Fold in the strawberries and chocolate chips.

Scoop out about ½ cup of batter into the heated skillet and spread it out into a 5-inch circle.

Cook for 5minutes until the edges start to cook and few bubbles begin to appear on top. Flip and cook for another 2-3 minutes. Repeat with the remaining batter until you have four large pancakes.

Serve with maple syrup and any toppings of choice.

Nutrition:

Energy (calories): 657 kcal

Protein: 24.35 g

Fat: 14.64 g

Carbohydrates: 108.83 g

7. Chocolate Coconut Vegan Energy Balls

Preparation Time: 20 minutes

Cooking Time: 20 minutes

Servings: 22 balls

Ingredients

¾ cup almonds – sliced or slivered

½ cup unsweetened cocoa

Two tablespoon ground flax seed

¼ teaspoon ground sea salt

1 1/3 cups organic old-fashioned rolled oats – gluten-free if desired

1 pound 16-ounce Medjool dates, pits removed

¼ cup unrefined coconut oil – melted

¼ cup finely shredded unsweetened coconut

Directions

Process the almond slice in a food processor for 20-30 seconds until finely chopped.

Add the cocoa, flaxseed, oats, and sea salt. Process for another 20 seconds until blended. Add dates and coconut oil and process for about 2 to 3 minutes until it's well blended. Form the mixture into balls (it should be sticky enough to form into balls). Place each ball into a plate or a baking sheet covered in parchment paper.

On a separate plate, add the finely shredded coconut. Press each ball, one at a time, into the coconut with a little pressure until it sticks to all sides. Transfer to an airtight container and store in the fridge for up to a week.

Nutrition: Calories: 59kcal| Carb: 6g| Protein: 2g| Fat: 3.6g|

8.   Ginger Greens Juice

Preparation Time: 5 minutes

Cooking Time: 15 minutes

Servings: 2

Ingredients

½ cup (120ml) water

1 (300g) cucumber

½ (80g) celery stalk

Two medium (375g) apples, seeded, halved

2 cups (60g) kale

One tablespoon (5g) fresh ginger root, peeled.

Directions:

Place all ingredients into the Vitamix container in the order listed and secure the lid. Select variable 1. Start the machine and slowly increase to its highest speed. Bled for 30 to 45 seconds, use the tamper to press the ingredients into the blades.

If using a programmed machine, press the smoothie button and allow the programmed cycle to complete.

Strain through a nut milk bag and store it in the refrigerator. Make sure you consume within two days.

Nutrition: Calories: 130kcal| Carb: 33g| Protein: 3g| Fat: 50g|

9. Tumeric Chicken & Kale Salad

Preparation Time: 20 minutes

Cooking Time: 30 minutes

Servings: 2

Ingredients

For The Chicken

250-300g 9-ounce chicken mince or diced up chicken thighs

One teaspoon ghee or one tablespoon coconut oil

½ medium brown onion, diced

One large garlic clove, finely diced

One teaspoon turmeric powder

½ teaspoon salt + pepper

One teaspoon lime zest

Juice of ½ lime

For The Salad

Six broccolini stalks or 2 cups of broccoli florets

Three large kale leaves stem removed and chopped

A handful of fresh coriander leaves, chopped

Two tablespoons pumpkin seeds (pepitas)

A handful of fresh parsley leaves, chopped

½ avocado, sliced

The Dressing

One small garlic clove, finely diced or grated

½ teaspoon wholegrain or Dijon mustard

½ teaspoon sea salt and pepper

Three tablespoons extra-virgin oil

Three tablespoons lime juice

One teaspoon raw honey

Directions:

Heat the coconut oil or ghee in a frying pan on medium-high. Add the onion and sauté on medium heat for 4-5 minutes, until golden. Add the chicken mince and the garlic heat for 2-3 minutes, stirring well.

Add the turmeric, lime juice, lime zest, pepper, and salt. Cook further for 3-4 minutes, stirring frequently. Set aside after it's cooked.

Meanwhile, while the chicken is cooking, bring a small saucepan of water to boil. Add the broccolini and cook for 2 minutes. Rinse (in cold water) and cut into 3 or 4 pieces.

Add the pumpkin seeds to the frying pan from the chicken and toast over medium heat for 2 minutes. Stir it frequently so that it won't burn.

Season with salt and set aside. You can also decide to use raw pumpkin seeds.

Place the chopped kale in a salad bowl and pour over the dressing. Toss and massage the kale with the sauce using your hands to soften the kale.

Finally, toss through the cooked chicken, broccolini, fresh herbs, pumpkin seeds, and avocado slices.

CHAPTER 2:

Lunch

10. Turmeric Chicken & Kale Salad

Preparation time: 10 minutes

Cooking time: 55 minutes

Servings: 4

Ingredients

For your poultry

1 tsp. ghee or one tablespoon coconut oil

1/2 moderate brown onion, diced

250 300 grams / 9 oz. Chicken mince or pops upward Chicken thighs

One large garlic clove, finely-manicured

1 tsp. turmeric powder

1teaspoon lime zest

juice of 1/2 lime

1/2 tsp. salt

For your salad

Six broccolini two or two cups of broccoli florets

two tbsp. pumpkin seeds (pepitas)

Three big kale leaves stalk removed and sliced

1/2 avocado, chopped

bunch of coriander leaves, chopped

couple of fresh parsley leaves, chopped

For your dressing table

3 tbsp. lime juice

One small garlic clove, finely diced or grated

3 tbsp. Extra-virgin Coconut Oil (I used 1. Tsp. avocado oil and 2 tbsp. EVO)

1 tsp. raw honey

1/2 tsp. Whole Grain or Dijon mustard

1/2 tsp. sea salt and salt

Directions:

Heat the ghee or coconut oil in a tiny skillet Pan above medium-high heat. Bring the onion and then sauté on moderate heat for 45 minutes, until golden. Insert the chicken blossom and garlic and simmer for 2-3 minutes on medium-high heat, breaking it all out.

Add the garlic, lime zest, lime juice, salt, and Soda and cook often stirring to get a further 3-4 minutes. Place the cooked mince aside.

As the chicken is cooking, make a little Spoonful of water. Insert the broccolini and cook for 2 minutes. Rinse under warm water and then cut into 3-4 pieces each.

Insert the pumpkin seeds into the skillet out of the Toast and chicken over moderate heat for two minutes, often stirring to avoid burning. Season with a little salt. Set aside. Raw pumpkin seeds will also be lovely to utilize.

Put chopped spinach in a salad bowl and then pour over the dressing table. With the hands, massage, and toss the carrot with the dressing table. It will dampen the lettuce, a lot similar to what citrus juice will not steak or fish carpaccio – it 'hamburgers' it marginally.

Finally, throw throughout the cooked chicken, Broccolini, fresh herbs, pumpkin seeds, and avocado pieces.

11.   Lamb, Butternut Squash And Date Tagine

Incredible Warming Moroccan spices create this balanced tagine perfect for cold autumn and chilly evenings. Drink buckwheat to get an excess overall health kick!

Preparation time: 10 minutes

Cooking time: 35 minutes

Servings: 4

Ingredients

2 Tsp. coconut oil

1 Red onion, chopped

2cm ginger, grated

3 Garlic cloves, crushed or grated

One teaspoon chili flakes (or to taste)

2 Tsp. cumin seeds

One cinnamon stick

Two teaspoons ground turmeric

800g lamb neck fillet, cut into 2cm chunks

1/2 Tsp. salt

100g Medjool dates, pitted and sliced

400g Tin chopped berries, and half of a can of plain water

500g Butternut squash, chopped into 1cm cubes

400g Tin chickpeas, drained

2 Tsp. fresh coriander (and extra for garnish)

Buckwheat, Cous-cous, flatbread, or rice to function

Directions

Pre Heat Your oven to 140C

Drizzle Roughly 2 tbsp. of coconut oil into a large ovenproof saucepan or cast-iron casserole dish. Add the chopped onion and cook on a gentle heat, with the lid for around five minutes, until the onions are softened but not too brown.

Insert The grated ginger and garlic, chili, cumin, cinnamon, and garlic. Stir well and cook for 1 minute off the lid. Add a dash of water when it becomes too humid.

Next, add from the lamb balls. Stir to coat the beef from the spices and onions, and then add the salt chopped meats and berries and roughly half of a can of plain water (100-200ml).

Bring the tagine to the boil, put the lid, and put on your skillet for about 1 hour and fifteen minutes.

Ten Moments before the conclusion of this cooking period, add the chopped butternut squash and drained chickpeas. Stir everything together, place the lid back and go back to the oven for the last half an hour of cooking.

When that, the tagine can removes from the oven and then stir fry throughout the chopped coriander. Drink buckwheat, couscous, flatbread, or basmati rice.

Notes

In case you do not have an ovenproof saucepan or cast iron casserole dish, then only cook the tagine at a standard saucepan until it must go from the oven and transfer the tagine to a routine lidded skillet before placing in the oven. Add in an additional five minutes of cooking time and energy to allow the simple fact that the noodle dish will probably be needing extra time to warm up.

12.   Prawn Arrabbiata-Sirtfood Recipes

Preparation time: 10 minutes

Cooking time: 25 minutes

Servings: 4

Ingredients

125-150 G Beef or cooked prawns (Ideally king prawns)

65 Gram Buckwheat pasta

1 Tablespoon Extra virgin coconut oil

To get the arrabbiata sauce

40 G Red onion, finely chopped

1 Garlic clove, finely chopped

30 Gram celery, thinly sliced

1 Bird's eye chili, finely chopped

1 Tsp. Dried mixed veggies

1 Tsp. extra-virgin coconut oil

2 Tablespoon White wine (optional)

400 Gram Tinned chopped berries

1 tbsp. Chopped parsley

Directions:

Fry the garlic, onion, celery, and peppermint and peppermint blossoms in the oil over moderate-low heat for 1--2 weeks. Turn up the heat to medium, bring the wine and cook 1 second. Add the berries and leave the sauce simmer over moderate-low heat for 20--half an hour, until it's a great creamy texture. If you're feeling that the sauce is becoming too thick, simply put in just a very little water.

While sauce is cooking, attract a bowl of water to the boil and then cook the pasta as per the package directions.

Once cooked to your dish, drain, then toss with the olive oil and also maintain at the pan before needed.

If you're utilizing raw prawns, put them into your sauce and cook for a further 3--four minutes, till they've turned opaque and pink, then add the parsley and function. If you're using cooked prawns, insert them using the skillet, and then bring the sauce to the boil, and then process.

Add the cooked pasta into the sauce, then mix thoroughly but lightly and function.

Nutrition:

Energy (calories): 168 kcal

Protein: 0.45 g

Fat: 18.15 g

Carbohydrates: 1.55 g

13. Turmeric Baked Salmon-Sirtfood Recipes

Preparation time: 10 minutes

Cooking time: 25 minutes

Servings: 4

Ingredients

125-150 Gram Skinned Salmon

1 Tsp. extra-virgin coconut oil

1 Tsp. Ground turmeric

1/4 Juice of a lemon

To get the hot celery

1 Tsp. extra-virgin coconut oil

40 G Red onion, finely chopped

60 Gram Tinned green peas

1 Garlic clove, finely chopped

1 Cm fresh ginger, finely chopped

1 Bird's eye chili, finely chopped

150 Gram Celery, cut into 2cm lengths

1 Tsp. darkened curry powder

130 Gram Tomato, cut into eight wedges

100 Ml vegetable or pasta stock

1 tbsp. Chopped parsley

Directions:

Heat the oven to 200C / gas mark 6

Start using the hot celery. Heat a skillet over moderate-low heat, and then add the olive oil, then the garlic, onion, ginger, celery, and peppermint. Fry lightly for two-three minutes until softened but not colored; you can add the curry powder and cook for a further minute.

Insert the berries afterward, your lentils and stock, and simmer for 10 seconds. You might choose to increase or reduce the cooking time according to how crunchy you'd like your sausage.

Meanwhile, mix the garlic olive oil and lemon juice and then rub the salmon. # Set on the baking dish and cooks for 8--10 seconds.

To complete, stir the skillet throughout the celery and function with the salmon.

14.   Coronation Steak Salad-Sirtfood Recipes

Preparation time: 20 minutes

Cooking time: 0minutes

Servings: 4

Ingredients

75 G Natural yogurt

Juice Of 1/4 of a lemon

1 Tsp. Coriander, sliced

1 Tsp. Ground turmeric

1/2 Tsp. darkened curry powder

100 G Cooked chicken, cut into bite-sized pieces

6 Walnut halves, finely chopped

1 Medjool date, finely chopped

20 G Crimson pumpkin, diced

1 Bird's eye illuminates

40 Gram Rocket, to function

Directions:

Mix the lemon, carrot juice, spices, and coriander in a bowl.

Add all of the remaining ingredients and serve on a bed of this rocket.

15.   Romaine Lettuce With Turmeric Potatoes

Preparation Time: 10 minutes

Cooking Time: 40 minutes

Servings: 4

Ingredients

600 g waxy potatoes

1tsp cumin seed

7 tbsp. virgin rapeseed oil

1tsp turmeric powder

120 ml of vegetable stock

3tbsp apple cider vinegar

salt

pepper

Two romaine lettuce hearts

100 g asparagus

Six stalks of parsley

1tsp black mustard seed

1tbsp breadcrumbs

6 tbsp. white wine vinegar

Four fresh eggsDirections:

Boil potatoes in boiling water for 15-20 minutes. Roast cumin in 1 tablespoon of hot oil while stirring. Stir in the turmeric, add the stock and vinegar, and bring to the boil. Salt and pepper broth vigorously. 4 tbsp. Of oil. Peel the potatoes cut them in half, and mix with the warm turmeric broth. Cover and let it soak for at least 1 hour.

Clean romaine lettuce, halved lengthways, and cut halves in 4 columns. Rinse emperor asparagus in a sieve and drain. Chop parsley leaves—heat two tablespoons of oil, roast mustard seeds in it, and stir in breadcrumbs.

Bring 1.5 l water to a boil with salt and vinegar. Beat the eggs one after the other in a soup spoon and slide them into the vinegar water. Using two forks lift the egg white over the egg yolk and shape it. Reduce heat. Let the eggs steep for 4-5 minutes. Arrange salad with asparagus and turmeric potatoes. Lift the eggs out of the broth, drain them briefly on kitchen paper, sprinkle with the crumbs, and arrange with the salad.

Nutrition:

Energy (calories): 1563 kcal

Protein: 25.42 g

Fat: 109.74 g

Carbohydrates: 123.56 g

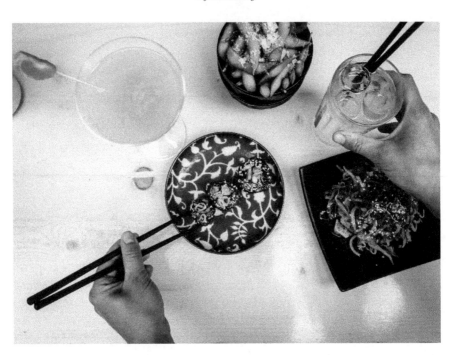

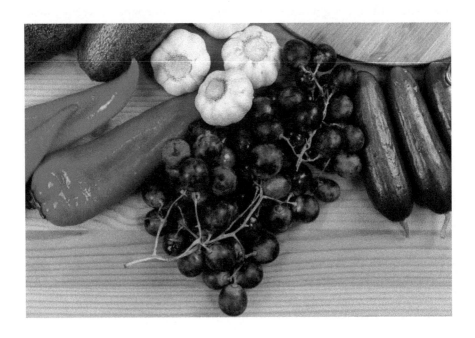

CHAPTER 3:

Dinner

16.   Quinoa Pilaf

Preparation Time: 30 minutes

Cooking Time: 20 minutes

Servings: 4 Servings

Ingredients

Two tablespoons extra virgin olive oil 1/2 medium yellow onion, finely chopped

1/4 bell pepper, finely chopped One garlic clove, minced Two tablespoons pine nuts

1 cup uncooked quinoa 2 cups of water Pinch freshly ground black pepper

Two tablespoons chopped fresh mint Two tablespoons chopped fresh basil or Thai basil*

One tablespoon chopped fresh chives (or green onions including the greens)

One small cucumber, peeled, seeds removed, chopped Salt and pepper

Directions:

Rinse the box with Directions: check your quinoa box. If you recommend washing it, place the quinoa in a large sieve and rinse it to remove water. (Some brands do not require washing). Onions, Peppers, garlic, pine nuts: Heat 1 tbsp. Put the olive oil over medium-high heat in a pot of 1/1 to 2 quarts. Add and cook onions, rusty peppers, garlic, and pine nuts, occasionally stirring until the onions are translucent but not browned. Add quinoa: add and cook uncooked quinoa, sometimes going for a few minutes.

You can toast a little quinoa for some bread. Add water, salt, stir: Add two glasses of water and a teaspoon of salt.

Bring to a boil and reduce heat so that cheese and water shine while the pot is partially covered (enough for steam). Cook for 20 minutes or until quinoa is thin and liquid is absorbed. Remove from heat and serve in a large bowl. Fill with a fork. Add olive oil, mint, basil, onion, and cucumber: add over low heat and add another tablespoon of olive oil. In chopped mint, mix basil, onion, and cucumber.

Add salt and pepper to taste. Chill or cool at room temperature.

Nutrition: Fat 22g, Carbohydrates 17g, and Protein 19g

17. Buckwheat And Mushroom Risotto

Preparation Time: 20 minutes

Cooking Time: 30 minutes

Servings: 6

Ingredients:

Black pepper, one teaspoon

Sea salt, one half teaspoon

Parsley, dried, one tablespoon

Buckwheat groats, four cups

Vegetable broth, two cups divided

Mushrooms, button, one cup sliced thin

Green bell pepper, one large, cleaned and minced

Red onion, one small, well diced

Capers, two teaspoons

Garlic, minced, two tablespoons

Marjoram, one teaspoon

Extra virgin olive oil, two tablespoons

Directions:

Fry the red onion, bell pepper, and garlic for five minutes.

Pour into the skillet one cup of the vegetable broth and the mushrooms and cook these for five more minutes.

Into this mixture, add the other cup of the vegetable broth and the buckwheat groats and cook all of this for ten minutes while stirring often. Pour in the capers, salt, pepper, and parsley and turn the heat under the pot to low.

Simmer this mixture for fifteen minutes or until the buckwheat groats are entirely cooked.

Nutrition:

Energy (calories): 2104 kcal

Protein: 8.56 g

Fat: 219.43 g

Carbohydrates: 49.76 g

18.   Halibut Chowder

Preparation Time: 20 minutes

Cooking Time: 70 minutes

Servings: 8

Ingredients:

Black pepper, one teaspoon

Extra virgin olive oil, one-fourth cup

Thyme, dried, one-fourth teaspoon

Tomato juice, one cup

Turmeric, one teaspoon

Basil, dried, one-half teaspoon

Sea salt, one-half teaspoon

Parsley, fresh, chopped, two tablespoons

Whole peeled tomatoes, two sixteen-ounce cans mashed with the juice

Garlic, minced, three tablespoons

Celery, three stalks chopped

Red onion, one medium peeled and chopped

Apple juice, one-half cup

Red bell pepper, one cleaned and chopped

Halibut steaks cut into cubes, three pounds

Directions:

Cook the celery, garlic, onion, and peppers in hot oil in a large soup pot for five minutes. Blend in the apple juice, herbs, mashed tomatoes, and tomato juice and stir everything together well. Simmer this mix for thirty minutes.

Drop the halibut pieces into the soup while stirring slowly. Add the pepper and salt and simmer for thirty more minutes.

Nutrition:

Energy (calories): 1036 kcal

Protein: 6.75 g

Fat: 94.33 g

Carbohydrates: 45.68 g

19.   Lamb Stew

Preparation Time: 25 minutes

Cooking Time: 70 minutes

Servings: 6

Ingredients:

Red wine, one-half cup

Parsley, fresh chop, three tablespoons

Turmeric, one teaspoon

Red bell pepper, one, seeded and chopped

Sea salt, one teaspoon

Zucchini, two small, peel, and slice

Lamb shoulder, boneless, two pounds cubed

Green beans, fresh, two cups trimmed

Potatoes, four, peeled and cubed

Oregano, dried, one teaspoon

Extra virgin olive oil, two tablespoons

Kale, chopped, one cup

Tomatoes, peeled and chopped, four cups

Chicken broth, one-half cup

Garlic, minced, three tablespoons

Black pepper, one teaspoon

Directions:

Sprinkle the salt and pepper on the lamb and cook it with the minced garlic in the hot oil in a large soup pot for five minutes. Mix in the broth and red wine and let this boil. Lower the heat and put in the oregano and tomatoes, stir everything together well and simmer for forty-five minutes.

Bring the soup back to an almost boil and stir in the red pepper, zucchini, green beans, and potatoes and cook for twenty more minutes while stirring often. Sprinkle the parsley on the soup to serve.

Nutrition: calories 389

20.   Celery And Smoked Sausage Soup

Preparation Time: 20minutes

Cooking Time: 70 minutes

Servings: 8

Ingredients:

- Thyme, crushed, one-half teaspoon

- Sea salt, one-half teaspoon

- Red onion, one chopped

- Extra virgin olive oil, one tablespoon

- Chicken broth, one cup

- Crushed tomatoes, one twenty-eight ounce can,

- Tomato sauce, one eight-ounce can

- Red beans, one fifteen ounces can mix with liquid

- Water, three cups

- Smoked sausage, one pound sliced

- Buckwheat groats, one-third cup uncooked

- Celery, six stalks diced

- Carrots, three diced

- Red chicory, one bunch, chopped

Directions:

Fry the red onion in the hot oil for five minutes. Stir the water and sausage into the pot. Add in the celery, carrots, crushed tomatoes, tomato sauce, beans, buckwheat groats, and chicory and mix everything well.

Mix in the bay leaf, salt, thyme, and broth. Boil all of this for one minute, and then lower the heat and let the soup simmer for one hour.

Nutrition: calories 404

CHAPTER 4:

Mains

21. Baked Potatoes With Spicy Chickpea Stew

Preparation time: 20 minutes

Cooking time: 2 hours

Servings: 12

Ingredients:

4-6 baking potatoes, pricked all over

tablespoons olive oil

red onions, finely chopped

cloves garlic, grated or crushed

2cm ginger, grated or finely cut into slices

½ -2 teaspoons chili flakes (probably depending on how hot and spicy you like your food)

Two tablespoons turmeric

Two tablespoons cumin seeds

Two tablespoons unsweetened cocoa powder (or cacao)

Splash of water

Two yellow peppers or green peppers (or whatever color you like!), chopped into bite-size pieces

2 x 400 g tins of chickpeas (or kidney beans, if you prefer) plus don't drain.

2 x 400g tins chopped tomatoes

Two tablespoons parsley plus extra for garnish

Salt and pepper to taste (optional)

Side salad (optional)

Directions:

Preheat the oven to 200°C while preparing all your ingredients.

When the oven is hot enough, place the baked potatoes in the oven and cook for 1 hour or until they're cooked like them.

When the potatoes cook in the oven, put the olive oil and diced red onion in a big broad saucepan and cook gently until the onions are soft but not dark.

Remove the cloth and add garlic, ginger, cumin, and chili. Cook on low heat for another minute, then add the turmeric and a relatively small splash of water, continue cooking for a minute, and take care that the plate is not dried.

Add onions, chocolate powder (or coffee), chickpeas (including chickpea water), and yellow pepper. Take to boil, then cook 45 minutes on low heat until thick and buttery (but don't let it burn!). The stew can be handled at the same time as potatoes.

Eventually, mix in 2 teaspoons of parsley and some salt and pepper; if needed, serve the stew over the baked potatoes or a small side salad.

22.   Bun-Less Beef Burgers With All The Trimmings

Preparation Time: 5 minutes

Cooking Time: 35 minutes

Servings: 4

Ingredients:

125 g Lean minced beef (5% fat)

15 g Red onion, finely chopped

1 tsp. Parsley, finely chopped

1 tsp. Extra virgin olive oil

150 g Sweet potatoes

1 tsp. Extra virgin olive oil

1 tsp. Dried rosemary

1 Garlic clove, unpeeled

10 g Cheddar cheese, sliced or grated

150 g Red onion, sliced into rings

30 g Tomato, sliced

10 g Rocket

1 Gherkin (optional)

Directions:

Let the temperature of over rising to 220°C / gas 7.

Start by making fries. Split the sweet potato into 1 cm thick slices. Add olive oil, rosemary, and garlic clove. Put on a baking sheet and fry for 30 minutes until good, crispy.

Combine the onion and parsley with the ground beef. Whether you have pastry cutters, mold your burger with the set's largest pastry cutter. Otherwise, just use your hands to produce an excellent even patty.

Steam a frying pan over medium heat, add olive oil, put the burger on one side of the pan, and rings on the other. Cook the burger on every side for 6 minutes, meaning it's finished.

Fry the onion rings to your taste.

When the burger is baked, add the cheese and red onion and melt the cheese in the hot oven for a minute.

Drop the onion, rocket, and gherkin. Serve the fries.

Nutrition:

Energy (calories): 379 kcal

Protein: 33.28 g

Fat: 13.02 g

Carbohydrates: 36.79 g

23. Chicken Skewers With Satay Sauce

Preparation Time: 5 minutes

Cooking Time: 25 minutes

Servings: 4

Ingredients:

150 g Chicken breast, cut into chunks

1 tsp. Ground turmeric

1/2 tsp. Extra virgin olive oil

50 g Buckwheat

30 g Kale, stalks removed and sliced

30 g Celery, sliced

4 Walnut halves, chopped, to garnish

20 g Red onion, diced

1 Garlic clove, chopped

1 tsp. Extra virgin olive oil

1 tsp. Curry powder

1 tsp. Ground turmeric

50 ml Chicken stock

150 ml Coconut milk

1 tbsp. Walnut butter or peanut butter

1 tbsp. Coriander, chopped

Directions:

Combine the chicken with the turmeric and olive oil and put it aside to marinate – it'd be better for 30 minutes to 1 hour, so if you're low on time, keep it as long as you can.

Cook the buckwheat with the container instructions, incorporating the kale and celery for the last 5–7 minutes of the cooking time. Wash.

Steam the barbecue at a high altitude.

Gently fry red onion and garlic in olive oil for 2–3 minutes until tender.

Add seasoning and cook another minute. Remove stock and coconut milk and curry to simmer, and then incorporate butter and whisk. Reduce heat and simmer for 8–10 minutes, or until smooth and soft.

Thread the chicken on the skewers and put under the hot grill for 10 minutes, rotating after 5 minutes.

Stir the coriander through the sauce, pipe over the skewers, and sprinkle over the sliced walnuts.

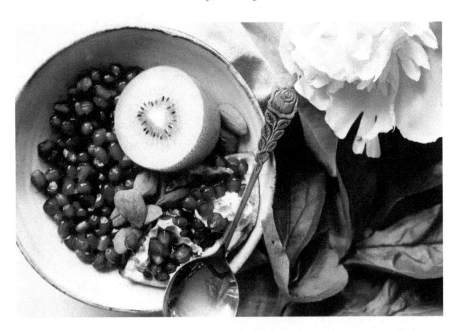

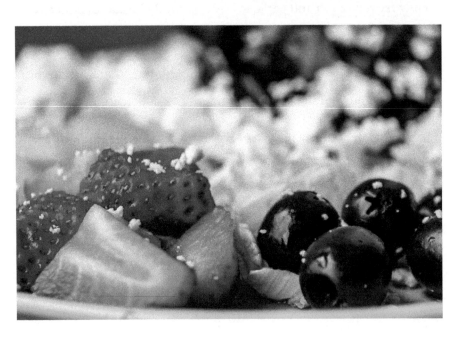

CHAPTER 5

Meat

24. Chicken And Kale Buckwheat Noodles

Preparation Time: 30 min.

Cooking Time: 25 minutes

Servings: 2

Ingredients:

For noodles

Finely chopped kale, 2 cup

Buckwheat noodles 5 oz.

Shiitake mushrooms (or any other of your choosing), four pieces

1 tsp. Extra virgin olive oil

One finely diced red onion

One diced chicken breast

One sliced bird's eye chili

Soy sauce 3 tbsp.

Salad dressing

Soy sauce, ¼ cup

Tamari sauce 1 tbsp.

Sesame oil 1 tbsp.

Lemon juice 1 tbsp.

Directions:

Boil or stir-fry chicken for up to 15 minutes.

Microwave kale for up to three minutes to preserve nutrients.

Cook buckwheat noodles and rinse and add kale once they're done.

Fry the mushrooms with 1 tsp. Of olive oil for up to three minutes and season with a pinch of salt. Set aside and use the same pan. Add more olive oil, sauté peppers, and chickpeas for up to five minutes. Add garlic, water, and tamari sauce, and cook for another three minutes. Add kale with noodles, chicken, and dressing. Mix all together and serve.

CHAPTER 6:

Sides

25.   Balsamic Vegetables With Feta & Almonds

Preparation Time: 5 minutes.

Cooking Time: 40 minutes

Servings: 4

Ingredients:

4 tbsp. olive oil

One red bell pepper, sliced

One green bell pepper, sliced

One orange bell pepper, sliced

½ head broccoli, cut into florets

Two zucchinis, sliced

Eight white pearl onions, peeled

Two garlic cloves halved

Two thyme sprigs, chopped

1 tsp. dried sage, crushed

2 tbsp. balsamic vinegar

Sea salt and cayenne pepper to taste

1 cup feta cheese, crumbled

½ cup almonds, toasted and chopped

Directions:

Preheat oven to 375 F. Mix all vegetables with olive oil, seasonings, and balsamic vinegar; shake well. Spread the vegetables out in a baking dish and roast in the oven for 40 minutes or until tender, flipping once halfway through. Remove from the oven to a serving plate. Scatter the feta cheese and almonds all over and serve.

Nutrition: Calories 276 Fat 23.3 g Carbs 7.9 g Protein 8.1 g

26. Stewed Vegetables

Preparation Time: 2 minutes.

Cooking Time: 30 minutes

Servings: 4

Ingredients:

2 tbsp. butter

One shallot, chopped

One garlic clove, minced

1 tsp. paprika

One carrot, chopped

Two tomatoes, chopped

One head cabbage, shredded

2 cups green beans, chopped

Two bell peppers, sliced

Salt and black pepper to taste

2 tbsp. parsley, chopped

1 cup vegetable broth

Directions:

Melt the butter in a saucepan over medium heat and sauté onion and garlic until fragrant, about 2 minutes.

Stir in bell peppers, carrot, cabbage, and green beans, paprika, salt, and pepper, add vegetable broth and tomatoes and cook on low heat for 25 minutes to soften. Serve sprinkled with parsley.

Nutrition: Calories 310 Fat 26.4 g Carbs 6 g Protein 8 g

CHAPTER 7:

Seafood

27. Asian Prawn Stir-Fry With Buckwheat Noodles

Preparation time: 10 minutes

Cooking time: 20 minutes

Servings: 4

Ingredients:

150 g of raw king prawns shelled, deveined

2 Tbsp. tamari (if you don't avoid gluten, you could use soy sauce)

2 Tbsp. virgin oil (extra olive oil)

Buckwheat noodles (75 g)

1 Clove of garlic, finely chopped

1 Chili, finely chopped

1 tsp. finely chopped fresh ginger

20g red onions, sliced

40g celery, trimmed and sliced

75g green beans, chopped

50g kale, roughly chopped

100ml chicken stock

5g celery leaves

Directions:

Set the frying pan over high heat, and then cook the prawns for 2–3 minutes in 1 teaspoon tamari and one teaspoon oil. Put the prawns onto a plate. Wipe the pan out of the oven with paper, because you will use it again.

Cook the noodles for 5–8 minutes in boiling water, or as directed on the packet. Drain and put away.

Meanwhile, over medium to high heat, fry the garlic, chili, ginger, red onion, celery, beans, and kale in the remaining oil for 2–4 minutes. Put the stock and bring to the boil, then cook for one or two minutes until the vegetables are cooked but crunchy.

Add the prawns, noodles, and leaves of lovage/celery to the pan, bring back to the boil, then remove the heat and serve.

28.   Baked Salmon Salad With Creamy Mint Dressing

Ingredients:

One salmon fillet (130g)

40g mixed salad leaves

40g young spinach leaves

Two radishes, trimmed and thinly sliced

50g of cucumber, cut into chunks

Two spring onions, trimmed and sliced

One small handful (10g) parsley, roughly chopped

For the dressing:

1 tsp. low-fat mayonnaise

1 tbsp. natural yogurt

1 tbsp. rice vinegar

Two leaves mint, finely chopped

Salt and brand new freshly black pepper

Directions:

Set the oven temperature to 200 ° C (180 ° C fan / Gas 6).

Place the salmon filet on a baking tray and bake for 18–20 minutes until it is just cooked. Switch off the oven, and then set aside. The salmon in the salad is equally good and hot or cold. Using a slice of fish, if your salmon has skin, just cook the skin side downwards and cut the salmon from the skin after cooking.

Mix the mayonnaise, yogurt, rice wine vinegar, mint leaves, and salt and pepper in a small bowl and leave to stand for at least 5 minutes to allow

Taste to grow.

Arrange on a serving plate the salad leaves, and spinach, and top with the radishes, the cucumber, the spring onions, and the parsley. Flake the cooked salmon over the salad and sprinkle over the dressing.

CHAPTER 8:

Poultry

29. Baked Chicken Breast With

Preparation time: 10 minutes

Cooking time: 65 minutes

Servings: 4

Ingredients:

15g parsley,

15g nuts,

15g of parmesan,

One tablespoon of extra virgin olive oil

1/2 lemon juice,

50ml of water,

150g of skinless chicken breast,

20g of red onions,

finely sliced,

One teaspoon of red wine vinegar,

35g arugula,

100g cherry tomatoes,

cut in half,

One teaspoon of balsamic vinegar.

Directions:

To prepare the pesto, put the parsley, walnuts, Parmesan cheese, and olive oil, half of the lemon juice, and a little water in a blender or food processor and blend until smooth. Add more water gradually until you have the consistency you prefer. Marinate the chicken breast in 1 tablespoon of pesto and the remaining lemon juice in the fridge for 30 minutes and even longer if possible. Heat the oven to 200°.

Heat a baking pan over medium-high heat. Fry the marinated chicken for 1 minute on each side, then transfer the pan to the oven and cook for 8 minutes or until cooked. Marinate the onions in red wine vinegar for 5-10 minutes. Drain the liquid.

When the chicken is cooked, take it out of the oven, pour another spoonful of pesto on top and let the heat of the chicken melt it. Cover with aluminum foil and leave to rest 5 minutes before serving. Mix arugula, tomatoes, and onions and sprinkle with balsamic vinegar. Serve with the chicken, pouring over the remaining pesto.

CHAPTER 9:

Vegetable

30.   Brussel Sprouts Croquettes

Preparation Time: 10 minutes

Cooking time: 25 minutes

Servings: 6

Ingredients:

Two eggs, beaten 1/3 cup coconut flour

One tablespoon flax meal ½ teaspoon salt

¾ cup fresh parsley, chopped

½ teaspoon ground black pepper

1 cup Brussel sprouts

Two eggs whisked

One tablespoon olive oil

2 cups water, for cooking

Directions:

Pour water into the pan. Add Brussel sprouts and close the lid.

Boil the vegetables for 15 minutes over medium heat.

After this, drain water and transfer Brussel sprouts into the blender.

Blend the vegetables until you get smooth mass.

After this, transfer Brussel sprout mass in the mixing bowl.

Add coconut flour, flax meal salt, chopped parsley, ground black pepper, eggs, and stir with the spoon's help until homogenous.

Pour olive oil into the skillet and preheat it.

Make the medium-sized croquettes from the vegetable mixture and cook them in the hot oil until golden brown.

Chill the croquettes a little and transfer them to the plates.

Nutrition: calories 87, fat 5.4, fiber 3.9, carbs 6.4, protein 4.2

31.   Vegetable Puree

Preparation Time: 10 minutes

Cooking time: 20 minutes

Servings: 3

Ingredients:

5 oz. celery root, peeled

One bell pepper

One garlic clove, peeled

One teaspoon avocado oil

¼ teaspoon salt

One teaspoon butter

1 cup water for cooking

Directions:

Remove the seeds from the bell pepper.

Place the celery root in the pan, add water, and bring it to a boil.

Boil the celery root for 15 minutes.

Then add bell pepper and switch off the heat.

Leave the vegetables for 2 minutes more in hot water.

After this, drain the water.

Add garlic, avocado oil, salt, and butter.

Use the hand blender to blend the vegetables into a puree.

The cooked puree will have a soft and smooth texture.

Nutrition: calories 47, fat 1.7, fiber 1.5, carbs 7.8, protein 1.2

32.   Curry Cauliflower Florets

Preparation Time: 10 minutes

Cooking time: 30 minutes

Servings: 4

Ingredients:

2 cups cauliflower florets

One tablespoon curry paste

½ cup of coconut milk

One egg whisked

1 cup coconut flakes

Directions:

Mix up together, whisk egg, curry paste, and coconut milk.

Then dip the cauliflower florets in the liquid and stir well.

Coat every cauliflower floret in the coconut flakes and transfer to the tray.

Preheat the oven to 360F.

Place the tray with the cauliflower florets in the oven and bake them for 30 minutes.

Flip the florets onto another side after 15 minutes of cooking.

Nutrition: calories 193, fat 17.2, fiber 3.7, carbs 8.5, protein 3.9

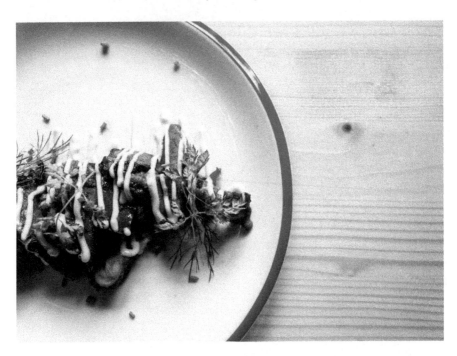

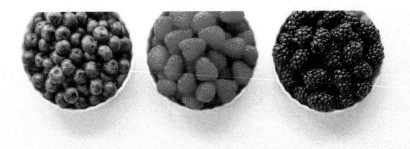

CHAPTER 10:

Soup, Curries and Stews

33. Kale Chicken Jambalaya

Preparation Time: 10 minutes

Cooking Time: 8 hours Servings: 8

Ingredients:

1 cup chopped onions & 2 minced garlic cloves

2 tbsp. Olive oil & 1 tsp. turmeric

Salt, black pepper to taste

3 pounds cubed chicken & 1 pound shrimp

1 tsp. dried red pepper flakes (to taste).

3 cups kale & 1 cup mushrooms

1 cup tomato paste & 1 cup chicken broth

1 cup corn & 1 cup chopped carrot

Direction:

Put ingredients in the slow cooker—cover & cook on low for 8 hours.

34. Kale, Quinoa And Beans Stew

Preparation Time: 10 minutes

Cooking Time: 7-9 hours

Servings: 8

Ingredients :

2 cups raw kidney beans

2 cups chopped onions

2 cups chopped kale

1 cup sliced carrot

2 tbsp. olive oil

2 cups tomatoes, chopped

Salt, black pepper, and ground cumin to taste

2 cups chicken or vegetable stock

1 cup quinoa

Direction:

Put ingredients in the slow cooker—cover & cook on low for 7 to 9 hours.

35.   Spicy Garbanzo And Kale Stew

Preparation Time: 10 minutes

Cooking Time: 7-9 hours

Servings: 8

Ingredients:

2 cups dry garbanzo beans

2 cups chopped onions

2 cups kale - 2 tbsp. olive oil

3 red peppers, chopped

2 cups tomato paste

Salt, ground cayenne pepper, and ground cumin to taste

2 cups chicken stock

4 pounds chicken meat

Direction:

Put ingredients in the slow cooker—cover & cook on low for 7 to 9 hours.

36.   Garbanzo Kale Curry

Preparation Time: 10 minutes

Cooking Time: 7-9hours

Servings: 8

Ingredients - Allergies: SF, GF, DF, EF, NF

4 cups dry garbanzo beans

Curry Paste, but go low on the heat

1 cup sliced tomato

2 cups kale leaves

1/2 cup coconut milk

Direction:

Put ingredients in the slow cooker—cover & cook on low for 7 to 9 hours.

Nutrition:

Energy (calories): 3065 kcal

Protein: 166.13 g

Fat: 48.89 g

Carbohydrates: 511.44 g

CHAPTER 11:

Snacks & Desserts

37.   Cream Cheese Stuffed Celery

Preparation Time: 15 minutes

Cooking Time: 25 minutes

Servings: 12

Ingredients:

Ten stalks celery, rinsed and dried well

16 oz. (2 packages) cream cheese softened to room temperature

One tablespoon milk

One ¼ oz. (1 packet) vegetable soup mix

½ cup walnut chips

½ cup bacon pieces, for topping

Directions:

Cut dried celery stalks into three sections each. Set aside. In a bowl, using an electric mixer, combine cream cheese and milk. Add dry vegetable soup mix and stir well.

Stuff the celery with cream cheese mixture. If your mixture is thin enough, you can use a piping bag with a tip and pipe the stuffing into the celery.

Sprinkle with walnut chips or bacon pieces (optional). Enjoy!

Nutrition: Calories 208 Fat 18g Carbohydrates 9g Protein 5g

38.   Baked Artichoke & Cilantro Pizza Dipping Sauce

Preparation Time: 10 minutes

Cooking Time: 28 minutes

Servings: 6

Ingredients:

1 – 6.5 oz. jar artichoke hearts, drained and chopped

½ cup pizza sauce, preferably with garlic

Two tablespoons fresh cilantro

¾ cup Parmesan cheese, grated

1/3 cup light mayonnaise

Garnish:

Fresh cilantro sprigs

Directions:

Heat oven to 350° F. Mix all of the dip ingredients together and spoon into a shallow ovenproof dish or 9-inch pie plate sprayed with non-stick cooking spray.

Bake 20 minutes until hot and bubbly.

Garnish with cilantro sprigs and serve warm. Serve with chips, nachos, bread, or veggies. Enjoy!

Nutrition: Calories 88 Fat 5g Carbohydrates 2g Protein 3g

39.   Herbed Soy Snacks

Preparation Time: 8 minutes

Cooking Time: 26 minutes

Servings: 16

Ingredients:

2 cups dry roasted soybeans

1 ½ teaspoons dried thyme, crushed

¼ teaspoon garlic salt

1/8 teaspoon cayenne pepper

Directions:

In a 15x10 inch baking pan, spread roasted soybeans in an even layer.

In a small bowl, combine thyme, garlic salt, and cayenne pepper. Sprinkle soybeans with thyme mixture—Bake in a 350° F oven for about 5 minutes or until heated through, shaking pan once. Cool completely, and enjoy!

Nutrition: Calories 75 Fat 3g Carbohydrates 4g Protein 7g

40.   Broccoli Cheddar Bites

Preparation Time: 15 minutes

Cooking Time: 20 minutes

Servings: 24

Ingredients:

One large bunch of broccoli florets

½ cup, packed, torn fresh bread

Two eggs, lightly beaten

¼ cup mayonnaise

¼ cup grated onion

1 ½ teaspoon lemon zest

1 cup packed, grated sharp cheddar cheese

¼ teaspoons freshly ground black pepper

½ teaspoon kosher salt

Directions:

Place it in 1 inch of water in a pot with a steamer basket. Bring to a boil. Add the broccoli florets. Steam the broccoli florets for 5 minutes, until just tender. Rinse with cold water to stop the cooking. Finely chop the steamed broccoli florets. You should have 2 to 2 ½ cups.

Place the beaten eggs and the cornbread in a large bowl. Mix until the bread is thoroughly moistened. Add the grated onion, mayonnaise, cheese, lemon zest, salt, and pepper. Stir in the minced broccoli.

Preheat the oven to 350° F. Coat the wells of 2 mini muffin pans with olive oil. Distribute the broccoli mixture in the muffin wells.

Bake at 350° F for 25 minutes until cooked through and lightly browned on top. If you don't have mini muffin pans, you can cook the bites freeform. Just grease a baking sheet and spoon large dollops of the mixture onto the pan. Baking time is the same.

Nutrition: Calories 62 Fat 4.8g Carbohydrates 3g Protein 1.7g

41.　No-Bake Zucchini Roll-Ups

Preparation Time: 10 minutes

Cooking Time: 20 minutes

Servings: 20

Ingredients:

One large zucchini

One jar pepperoncini

One medium carrot

Handful mixed greens

One tub guacamole

One single celery stalk

Fresh dill

Directions:

You were using a peeler to slice the zucchini in a long way on all sides to avoid the center. Basically, make 3-4 slices on one side and move on to the opposite side, then the other two sides until you have about 20 pieces. Don't discard the middle; just add to your next skillet meal. Set aside.

Using the mandolin slicer, cut the carrots and celery into thin strips and set aside.

Finally, cut the top part off each pepperoncino and cut it on one side to open and clean the seeds out.

Arranging the Roll-Ups:

On a flat surface, place one zucchini stip. Spread a dab of guacamole on one end. Place a pepperoncino on top of the guacamole, open side up. Fill the pocket whole of the pepperoncini with guacamole. Add in 1-2 mixed green leaves, three strips of carrots, 1-2 strips of celery, fresh dill, and roll it tight until you reach the end of the zucchini. If you need help keeping the zucchini roll-ups close in place, add another dab of guacamole on the end part of the zucchini to stick together.

Do this step until you've used all the ingredients.

Serve cold and refrigerate leftover for up to 24 hours. The guacamole will darken after this time.

Nutrition: Calories 214 Fat 4.7g Carbohydrates 4g Protein 5g

42. Spicy Deviled Eggs

Preparation Time: 15 minutes

Cooking Time: 15 minutes

Servings: 24

Ingredients:

12 large eggs

One tablespoon Sriracha sauce

1/3 cup mayonnaise

One tablespoon Dijon mustard

Fine chili flakes

Fresh chives, minced

Salt and freshly ground black pepper to taste

Directions:

Fill a saucepan with enough water to cover eggs by an inch and bring to a full boil. Carefully lower eggs into boiling water.

Let eggs cook uncovered for about 30 seconds. Reduce heat to low and cover.

 Simmer for 11 minutes.

Transfer boiled eggs to a bowl of ice water. When cool enough to handle, gently break the shell apart and peel. If possible, refrigerate eggs overnight, making them easier to cut.

Once eggs are cold, cut them in half lengthwise with a very sharp knife. Carefully spoon yolks out into a small bowl and arrange whites on a serving platter. In a medium bowl, mash yolks into a paste with the back of a fork. Add mayonnaise, Sriracha sauce, and mustard; whisk until smooth. Season it to taste with salt, freshly ground black pepper, and more Sriracha if you like. Spoon or pipe the filling into egg white halves.

Cover and refrigerate eggs for 2 hours or more (up to 1 day). Once chilled, sprinkle generously with fine chili flakes and minced chives. Serve and enjoy!

Nutrition: Calories 53 Fat 4g Net Carbs 0.6g Protein 2 g

CHAPTER 12:

Desserts

43.   Strawberry Rhubarb Crisp

Preparation Time: 10 minutes

Cooking Time: 45 minutes

Servings: 8

Ingredients:

1 cup white sugar

½ cup buckwheat flour + 3 tbsp.

3 cups strawberries, sliced

3 cups rhubarb, diced

½ lemon, juiced

1 cup packed brown sugar

1 cup coconut oil, melted

¾ cup rolled oats

¼ cup buckwheat groats

¼ cup walnuts, chopped

Directions:

Preheat the oven to 375 ° F. In a large bowl, mix the white sugar, 3 tbsp. Flour, strawberries, rhubarb, and lemon juice. Place the mixture on a 9-by-13-inch baking sheet.

In a separate bowl, mix ½ cup of flour, brown sugar, coconut oil, oats, buckwheat groats, and walnuts until crumbly.

Crumble over the rhubarb and strawberry mixture. Bake 45 minutes in the preheated oven, or until crisp and lightly browned.

Nutrition: Calories 167 Fat 3.1 g Carbohydrate 58.3 g Protein 3.5 g

44. Maple Walnut Cupcakes With Matcha Green Tea Icing

Preparation Time: 20 minutes

Cooking Time: 25 minutes

Servings: 24

Ingredients:

For the Cupcakes:

2 cups of All-Purpose flour

½ cup buckwheat flour

2 ½ teaspoons baking powder

½ tsp. salt

1 cup of cocoa butter

1 cup white sugar

1 tbsp. pure maple syrup

Three eggs

2/3 cup milk

¼ cup walnuts, chopped

For the Icing:

3 tbsp. coconut oil, thick at room temperature

3 tbsp. icing sugar

1 tbsp. Matcha green tea powder

½ tsp. vanilla bean paste

3 tbsp. cream cheese softened

Directions:

Preheat the oven to 350 degrees F. Place paper cups in muffin cups for 24 regular sized muffins. In a medium bowl, combine the flours, baking powder, and salt.

In a separate large bowl, mix the sugar, butter, syrup, and eggs with a mixer. Add to dry ingredients, rearrange, and add milk.

Pour the batter into the muffin cup until 2/3 full.

Cook for 20-25 minutes or until an inserted toothpick comes out clean.

Cool completely before frosting.

To make the icing: Add the coconut oil and powdered sugar to a bowl and use a hand mixer to whisk until clear and smooth.

Mix in the matcha powder and vanilla. Finally, add the cream cheese and beat until smooth. Pipe or spread them on the cupcakes once they are cold.

Nutrition: Calories 164 Fat 6 g Carbohydrate 21 g Protein 2 g

45.   Green Tea Smoothie

Preparation Time: 10 minutes

Cooking Time: 3minutes

Servings: 2

This super healthy smoothie uses an incredibly enriched Japanese green tea blended with matcha powder. It is accessible in Asian specialists or tea shops.

Ingredients:

250 of ml milk

Two ripe bananas

1/2 tsp. of vanilla bean paste (not extract) or a small scrape of the seeds from a vanilla pod

2 tsp. of matcha green tea powder

2 tsp. of honey

Six ice cubes

Direction:

  Simply mix every ingredient in a mixer, processor, or blender and serve in two cups.

Nutrition: Energy (calories): 184 kcal Protein: 1.31 g Fat: 5.85g

Carbohydrates: 35.15 g

46.   Sirt Food Miso Marinated Cod

Preparation Time: 10 minutes

Cooking Time: 30 minutes

Servings: 1

Ingredients:

1tbsp of mirin

20g miso

200g of skinless cod fillet

1tbsp of extra virgin olive oil

40g of celery, sliced

20g red onion, sliced

1bird's eye chili, finely chopped

One garlic clove, finely chopped

60g green beans

1tsp of finely chopped fresh ginger

1 tsp. of sesame seeds

50g kale, roughly chopped

1tbsp of tamari

5g parsley, roughly chopped

1 tsp. of ground turmeric

30g buckwheat

Directions:

Mix the miso, mirin, and one teaspoon of olive oil. Clean the entire cod, apply the mix, and set for 30 minutes to marinate. To 220oC / gas fire the oven to 7.

Ten minutes to bake cod.

Heat a wide frying bowl in the meantime or wok with the rest of the oil. Add the celery, garlic, curry, ginger, green beans, and kale, and then leave it for a few minutes. Tender fry until it is cooked. To help the cooking phase, you can have to apply a little water to the oven.

Cook the buckwheat with the turmeric for 3 minutes according to the package directions.

Serve in a stir fry with greens and shrimp; incorporate sesame seeds, parsley, tamari.

47. Raspberry And Blackcurrant Jelly-Sirt Food Recipes

Preparation Time: 10 minutes

Cooking Time: 15 minutes

Servings: 2

Jelly-making is an ideal way to prepare the fruit such that it can consume in the morning for the first time.

Ingredients:

Two leaves of gelatin, Sirtfood recipes

100g raspberries, washed

Two tbsp. of granulated sugar

100gm blackcurrants washed and stalks removed

300ml of water

Directions:

Arrange in two dishes/glasses/mold the raspberries. In a bowl of cold water, soften the gelatin leaves.

Put in sugar and 100ml of water and use to boil the blackcurrants in a small pot. Drop in to the fire and whisk vigorously for five minutes. Wait for two minutes.

Spray the gelatin leaves with extra water and add it to the pot. Add the remaining water until it is dissolved. Put the fluid in the cooked plates and cool to set. In 3-4 hours or overnight, the jellies should be placed.

Nutrition: calories 76

48.   Apple Pancakes With

Preparation Time: 10 minutes

Cooking Time: 20 minutes

Servings: 4

These pancakes are healthy and decadent. A lovely morning dish

Ingredients:

75g of porridge oats

2 tbsp. of caster sugar

1tsp of baking powder

125g plain flour

Two apples, peeled, cored, and cut into small pieces

Pinch of salt

Two egg whites

300ml of semi-skimmed milk

2 tsp. of light olive oil

For the compote:

2 tbsp. of caster sugar

120g of blackcurrants, washed and stalks removed

3 tbsp. of water

Directions:

Make the compote first. Put the blackcurrants, sugar, and water in a small saucepan. Bring to a burner and boil for 10-15 minutes.

In a wide pot, put the oats, flour, baking powder, caster sugar, and salt and mix well. Stir in the apple and whisk in the milk a little at a time until you have a smooth blend. Whisk the egg whites to firm peaks, then insert them into the batter for the pancake. Put the batter over to a jug.

Heat 1/2 tsp. of oil over medium-high heat in a non-stick frying pan and dump around one-fourth of the batter into it. Cook until light brown on all sides. Do the same for the four pancakes and repeat to make.

Eat the pancakes drizzled over with blackcurrant compote.

Nutrition: calories 377

49.   Fruit Salad

Preparation Time: 10 minutes

Cooking Time: 10 minutes

Servings: 1

This fruit salad is filled with the finest SIRT fruits.

Ingredients:

1tsp of honey

½ cup of freshly made green tea

One apple, cored and roughly chopped

One orange halved

Ten blueberries

Ten red seedless grapes

Directions:

Stir in half a cup of green tea with the sugar. When diluted, add the half orange juice. Leave on to cool down.

Cut the other half of the orange and put the sliced fruit, grapes, and blueberries together in a dish. Pour over the cooled tea, and leave too steep before serving for a few minutes.

Nutrition:Energy (calories): 121 kcal Protein: 0.75 g Fat: 0.32 g

Carbohydrates: 31.87 g

50. Bites-Sirt Food Recipes

Preparation Time: 10 minutes

Cooking Time: 30 minutes

Servings: 4

Ingredients

30g of dark chocolate (85 percent cocoa solids), broken into pieces; or cocoa nibs

120g of walnuts

1tbsp of cocoa powder

250g Medjool dates, pitted

1tbsp of extra virgin olive oil

1 tbsp. of ground turmeric

1–2 tbsp. of water

the scraped seeds of one vanilla pod or 1 tsp. of vanilla extract

Directions:

In a food processor, place the walnuts and chocolate and process them until they make a fine powder. Add all the remaining ingredients except water and combine until the mixture forms a disk. Depending on the paste's strength, you may or do not have to apply the water-you don't want it to be so wet.

Shape the mixture into bite-sized balls with your hands and refrigerate in an airtight jar for at least one hour before feeding.

Add in some more chocolate or desiccated cocoa. You could roll any of the balls to obtain a different finish if you want.

They'll stay in your fridge for up to one week.

Nutrition:

Energy (calories): 1752 kcal

Protein: 27.08 g Fat: 98.43 g

Carbohydrates: 227.11 g

Conclusions

Most diets have been proven to be just a temporary fix. If you want to keep weight off for a good while maintaining muscle mass and ensuring that your body stays healthy, then you need to be following a diet that activates your sirtuin genes: in other words, the Sirtfood Diet.

You should also ensure you have a green sirtfood-rich juice every day to get all of those sirtuins- activating ingredients into your body. Also, feel free to indulge in tea, coffee, and the occasional glass of red wine. And most importantly, be adventurous. Now is the time to start leading a happy, healthy, and fat-free life without having to deprive you of delicious and satisfying food.

Lightning Source UK Ltd.
Milton Keynes UK
UKHW020828180321
380564UK00005B/40